OPTICIAN TRAINING

*How to increase your eyewear sales
and turnover in 13 steps*

CHRISTIAN MÜLLER

Copyright 2019 - All rights reserved.

The purpose of this document is to provide accurate and reliable information on the subject and topics covered. The publication is sold with the understanding that the publisher is not required to provide any accounting, regulatory or other qualified services. If legal or professional advice is required, a person practising this profession should be appointed.

- From a policy statement adopted and approved by a committee of the American Bar Association and a committee of publishers and associations alike.

It is in no way legal to reproduce, duplicate or transmit parts of this document in electronic or printed form. The recording of this publication is strictly prohibited and any storage of this document is only permitted with the written permission of the publisher. All rights reserved.

The information provided herein is truthful and consistent, as any liability for carelessness or otherwise by the use or misuse of any policies, processes or instructions contained herein is the sole and complete responsibility of the recipient's reader. In no event shall the Publisher be liable, directly or indirectly, for any repair, damage or loss arising out of or in connection with the information contained herein.

The author owns all copyrights not owned by the publisher.

The information contained herein is provided for informational purposes only and is therefore universal. The information is presented without contract or warranty of any kind.

The trademarks used are without consent and the publication of the trademark is without permission or support by the trademark owner. All trademarks and brands in this book are for informational purposes only and belong to the owners themselves and are not associated with this document.

This book contains the author's opinions and ideas and is intended to provide people with helpful and informative knowledge. The strategies it contains may not suit every reader, and there is no guarantee that they will work for everyone. The use of this book and the implementation of the information contained therein is expressly at your own risk. The author cannot assume liability for any damages of any kind for any legal reason.

Liability claims against the author for material or immaterial damage caused by the use or non-use of information or by the use of incorrect and/or incomplete information are generally excluded. The work including all contents was compiled with the greatest care. However, the author does not guarantee the topicality, correctness, completeness and quality of the information provided. Misprints and misinformation cannot be completely excluded. The author cannot assume any legal responsibility or liability in any form for erroneous information and the resulting consequences.

Dedication

My family and my friends, who always support me at all times.

THIS BOOK WILL HELP YOU:

to find new ways of striving for new goals in sales

*

to win customers faster and easier

*

to win customers for their thoughts

*

to entertain your customers for your eyeglasses

*

to increase your persuasiveness, reputation and communication skills.

*

to improve your position in sales and maximize your turnover

CONTENT

Introduction 1

1. 12 Steps Before the Sales Success 7

2. Only Those Who Know Their Goal Can Achieve It 19

3. The Probably Best Paid Quality In The World 29

4. How To Create Sympathy To The Customer Through Mirroring 35

5. Recognize Types Of Buyers 41

6. NLP - Convincing In The Language Of The Customer 49

7. Benefit-Instead Characteristic Reasoning 59

8. Women Buy Differently from Men 65

9. The 3-Glasses-Rule 75

10. First Give, Then Take 79

11. Color - And Type Consulting 85

12. How To Open Sales Talks For Which You Will Love Your Customers 93

13. Know Buy Signals, Use Deal Techniques And Sell! 97

8 TIPS ON HOW TO GET THE MOST OUT OF THIS BOOK:

1. Have the sincere and burning desire to master the skills of dealing with clients.

2. Read each topic twice before moving on to the next one.

3. Pause reading more often and think about how to put the advice into practice in your case.

4. Take notes and mark important sentences.

5. Review the book every month.

6. Use the methods contained therein at every opportunity.

7. Note your progress every week and consider what successes you have achieved, what mistakes you have made and how you can do better in the future.

8. Write down how and when you acted according to the methods.

INTRODUCTION

"Where your interest is, there's your energy."
~ Dale Carnegie

My heart pounded. I stood there nervously and stiffly, as if I had to give a biology lecture in front of a school class, without even knowing the slightest thing about the topic being asked for.

It was the first day of my training as an optician and I was now standing behind a long counter in the spacious sales room of the modern and stylishly furnished shop. There were 15 customers romping around in the room.

The sun was at its zenith. The whole sales stage was brightly lit. My new colleagues were immediately in their element and I saw how they handled the customers with full eagerness to their new glasses.

It was a picture like in a discotheque, where the thirsty guests quickly go to the bar and serve their cooling drink, only with the difference that our guests demanded convincing advice!

Since all colleagues were now busy with the customers thirsting for advice, I was thrown as a newbie immediately into the known cold water and had to watch to serve the customers remaining for me well.

I bundled all my energy and confidence, greeted the strangers friendly and started to find out what kind of glasses they wanted.

As a fresh high school graduate, without experience in sales, I naturally had no red thread, no knowledge of glasses and little idea of advice. Now I should fulfill a whole day long shoppinglustigen humans their eyeglass desires, since except me all further colleagues were likewise busy with it.

To cut a long story short: I managed to sell a few pairs of glasses, but in the end it was certainly more sympathy values than sales masterpieces that motivated the customers to buy.

Because more than my energy and endurance, I didn't have to offer the customers on this day.

The next day I saw myself in another shop of my new training company. The noble and comfortable furnishing received the particularly demanding customers.

And what fascinated me on this day still fascinates me today! My task was to give me a broad overview of the dazzling assortment of glasses and to observe my new colleagues at the same time. Fortunately for me, the talented managing director received his first customer and the stage was clear for his appearance.

He was immediately in a familiar conversation with this stranger, laughed with her, used confident and carefully chosen words, and managed to entertain the customer, inspire him and awaken the unequivocal desire for a particular pair of glasses.

I have never seen such a great consultation before! The client's big eyes and relaxed posture revealed that he had apparently never experienced anything like it before. The customer was captured as if in an exciting film by the words he heard from the managing director. At that moment my boss at that time not only awakened the astonished customer's desire for a certain pair of glasses, but also my burning desire to become an expert optician during my consultation! I wanted to manage to make the customer's eyes shine, while I arouse the need for glasses in him with full motivation and the most eye-catching pictures.

For me the decision was made to learn everything imaginable and useful about the successful consultation in order to be able to apply it effectively.

This is where my path began, dear reader. A way where the nights got longer to read the numerous books about consulting and sales.

A path that led me to exciting sales training courses and allowed me to learn from professional role models.

A direction full of new and useful insights that I got because I was looking for them. My hunger for this knowledge was so great that I also had to think outside the box of my own industry, so that I gained even more experience through the methods of other industries in order to be able to advise even more successfully.

A very tedious and costly way, from which you can profit now shortly.

At the beginning of my career as a consultant in ophthalmic optics, I would have wished for such a book.

A book that immediately delivers proven procedures in the sale of ophthalmic optics as well as shows the latest and cross-industry methods in convincing customer consulting.

What you hold in your hands and see in front of you is a collection of the most useful and effective methods to inspire customers for your product in ophthalmic optics and to multiply your turnover.

A treasure chest full of tried and tested instruments to present you and your product in the right light on the sales stage. A buffet from which you take exactly what you need for the respective situation.

In addition, you invest in the most effective and cheapest advertising for yourself and your business: your customers!

For me the decision was made to learn everything imaginable and useful about the successful consultation in order to be able to apply it effectively.

This is where my path began, dear reader. A way where the nights got longer to read the numerous books about consulting and sales.

A path that led me to exciting sales training courses and allowed me to learn from professional role models.

A direction full of new and useful insights that I got because I was looking for them. My hunger for this knowledge was so great that I also had to think outside the box of my own industry, so that I gained even more experience through the methods of other industries in order to be able to advise even more successfully.

A very tedious and costly way, from which you can profit now shortly.

At the beginning of my career as a consultant in ophthalmic optics, I would have wished for such a book.

A book that immediately delivers proven procedures in the sale of ophthalmic optics as well as shows the latest and cross-industry methods in convincing customer consulting.

CHRISTIAN MÜLLER

What you hold in your hands and see in front of you is a collection of the most useful and effective methods to inspire customers for your product in ophthalmic optics and to multiply your turnover.

A treasure chest full of tried and tested instruments to present you and your product in the right light on the sales stage. A buffet from which you take exactly what you need for the respective situation.

In addition, you invest in the most effective and cheapest advertising for yourself and your business: your customers!

CHAPTER 1

12 STEPS BEFORE THE SALES SUCCESS

"Do you love life? Then don't waste any time, because that's what life is all about!" ~ *Benjamin Franklin*

When I look back on my initial time as a trainee, I am always amazed at the little things that changed the course. As I already reported in the introduction, I decided to continue by studying various books on the sale. There was an enormous offer on the subject of sales and advice. My favourite thing would have been to order a dozen of these helpful books and to wrap them up like a hungry dog standing in front of a big bowl full of juicy treats.

Since my financial means as a trainee were of course limited and I had to determine first of all which knowledge really leads me to success, I researched.

So in the evening I found myself busy on the internet finding out what methods successful people use in their lives. What kind of recipes do you use to conjure up your six-star menus?

How do the most successful people of our time use their inner navigator to reach their goals most effectively and effectively? Is there such a thing as a certain system that you have acted upon to see success? Or do they simply always have luck, inheritances or an above-average IQ?

I can reassure you, because there is a certain way of acting that makes these people winners! For this I read biographies of famous personalities like Benjamin Franklin and looked for mentors who understood how to lead other people to their success.

The best examples are the coaches of professional athletes. Professional athletes manage to achieve exactly the goal they demand from themselves through a certain sequence of their actions. Therefore I studied books of the most important and influential coaches so that I could best program my personal navigation system.

What I found out after my extensive and exciting research you can see in the following steps!

The secret of the people who achieve their goals lies in the fact that they set their goals and do exactly what brings them closer to their goals. Since my success also began with acting exactly according to these steps, it is probably also particularly important for your success to learn this knowledge first.

One:

They must have a great hunger, a strong need and an irrepressible desire for a certain goal! So ask yourself what you want to be, do or have. Which wish would inspire you the most if you knew that you could reach it?

Which goal fills you with pride and satisfaction? The strength of your personal need determines the strength and the unlockedness with which you strive for your goal.

Secondly:

You must be convinced that you can achieve your desired goal! So believe that you will learn the skills and qualities necessary to achieve your wish! Successful people have always had a strong belief that they will achieve what they want.

Benjamin Franklin ⊠s It was his belief in the independence of states that drove him to draft the Declaration of Independence together with a few other political supporters. The danger of going to British prison for it was all present. Only his belief in the realization of this goal helped him to overlook his fear in order to create something from which the people of the USA still profit today.

The wonderful thing is that every day you work towards something, your faith and your conviction become stronger and stronger.

In order to stay motivated and rejoice in success, you should divide your goal into smaller milestones.

Therefore, set realistically achievable stage goals at the beginning, which you then tick off from your list. This approach keeps you on a strongly motivating course for success and you feel more and more self-confident from day to day.

This build-up of self-esteem is very important so that you have a very specific attitude towards further challenging goals. The attitude of being able to create an even bigger goal!

Thirdly:

Write down your goal! A few years ago, Dr. Karan Horney conducted a study in which the test persons were taught how to set goals. The subjects wrote down their goals and the results were pro- tocolated over months and years. The fantastic result of this study was that 95 percent of the participants achieved their goals.

A motivating result, wasn't it? Successful people work with detailed plans and review their actions daily. I therefore recommend that you write down your goals anew every day so that you can reach your subconsciousness and thus provide the right impetus. Ask yourself again and again how you can get closer to your goal and write it down.

Four:

In the fourth step you determine your starting point. For example, if you want to sell a certain number of sunglasses per month, first write down how many you have currently sold per month. This step is important for you, as it gives you an overview of how many sunglasses you have sold per month and how many you are missing from your current point to your target sales. In addition, you set yourself realistic goals from the outset, because you have honestly grasped your starting point and can thus increase sales step by step, instead of never getting the situation through unrealistic wishes.

Fifth:

In the fifth step, you visualize all the reasons why you have chosen this goal. Personally, I enjoy this part very much, because I keep in mind why I actually chose this goal.

It's very motivating to see what you can have, do or be after reaching your goal. Write down as many reasons as possible, because they act like petrol in your engine and provide the right drive.

Sixth:

Just like trains have a departure schedule, after which they start and arrive, you set a time when you want to have reached your destination. It is very advantageous to set a time limit. You will be more motivated and discipled to hold out even under adverse circumstances, because you know that your goal will be reached in the near future and you can then be very proud of yourself.

After I started to set my goals in all spheres of life, I was motivated to achieve them within the time frame. Of course there were also difficulties in reaching my goals, but I solved them easier and faster, because I always had my time to reach the goal in mind. Therefore, write down the goal at which you want to have achieved your goal and let it spur you on!

Seventhly:

A big difference between successful and unsuccessful people is that successful people ask themselves what prevents them from not having what they want. They think about what inner obstacles or blockages they have, which block their way to the goal. They do not blame other people or other circumstances, but remove the snow in front of their own house so that they can walk unhindered along the path.

So it is essential that you now write down what is currently preventing you from having achieved what you want.

Eighth:

To reach your goal, write down what information, what features, and what skills you need to achieve them. Never before have there been so many possibilities as today to obtain a great deal of valuable information from the most diverse areas of life. In today's world, in which knowledge and not capital or social status is important, everyone has the chance to have a lot of success.

You have certainly heard of the young student who, with his knowledge of computer science and a few other students, founded an Internet company in 2004, which within a few years became an empire estimated at around 50 billion US dollars today.

Right, we're talking about Mark Zuckerberg and Facebook. So you can see how knowledge about a certain area can give you the chance to achieve great success.

Ninth:

Just as Mark Zuckerberg needed support from his young partners, you will now benefit greatly if you consider who you can cooperate with in the future so that you can achieve your goal quickly. Think about who can support you from your environment and also consider how you can help the others so that you earn their help. You will reach your goal faster and better if you cultivate more and better relationships. You will live later in the book with me, as I manage through relationships to be able to attend free seminars of high-ranking companies about the sale, which would have cost on the free market several hundred euros.

Make a note of which people are the most important in your private and professional life. Which person could become important for you in the future?

Tenthly:

If you want to get into a car and drive from Berlin to Zurich, it is very useful for you to switch on the navigation system and enter your destination. The navigation system will then calculate in advance which route is best for you so that you can reach your destination as quickly as possible. You therefore drive according to a plan. So that you can reach your professional destination in the best possible way, be your own navigation system. Make a note of what you need to do first and second. Which abilities, skills and information do you have to learn one after the other in order to reach your destination successfully? Determine how you divide your days, weeks and months.

For example, if you intend to sell a certain number of glasses in a certain period of time, you can distribute the number among weekly, daily and monthly targets. Achieving these goals will increase your self-esteem and make you feel positive and energetic. So let yourself be inspired by the successful strategy of setting milestones and learning the knowledge that will bring you closer to your goal.

Eleven:

Setting this part of the goal is probably the best! The best way to do this is to find a relaxed place to play in your apartment. Now visualize in your imagination how you have just reached your goal and imagine the situation as lively as possible.

See how you are pleased about the desired result and what a positive feeling you experience.

Feel how happy and satisfied you will be and how proud the desired situation makes you.

It is best to use all your senses. Imagine how you reach your goal, hear how you are happy about it and feel the beautiful feelings you experience. It is best to repeat this exercise in the morning and in the evening so that this goal drives and motivates you more and more.

Twelfth:

In this last step you decide for yourself to pursue your goal resolutely. Take on the task of doing what you need to do. Perform infallibly what you set out to do. This decision is of great importance for you, because it enables you to hold out even in difficult situations and to master challenges better. The valuable things in life are often not easy to get. But if you manage to hold out, then success is guaranteed.

Benjamin Franklin, one of the most important scientists and inventors of the world, could have written about his numerous great inventions in his biography, but instead he wanted to leave something much more important to mankind. Thus he wrote in his book mainly about his twelve rules to lead a contented and successful life. One of these rules states that we should act decisively and do what is necessary to achieve our goal.

Let this wisdom inspire you and start right away. Create a folder where you can file your lists with your goals, plans, etc.

Start now and write on a sheet of paper your eight most important goals you want to achieve in the next six to twelve months. Describe your goals as if you had already achieved them.

As an example, you can write, "I sell ten pairs of glasses a day."

Now take the goals and go through each one after the twelve steps. Think about which of the goals have the highest priority for you and tackle them immediately. Just writing down the goals will put you in a positive and motivating state, as you will have clarity about your wishes. It is also important that you start immediately to set yourself stage goals and take the first steps to achieve them.

If you have the urge for success in your profession and want to be one of the best in your field, then learn from one of the best methods to achieve your goals quickly and effectively. You will feel how you feel better from day to day by working towards your goals. You will see yourself getting closer to your desires and hear more and more the inner voice saying:

"Soon I have reached my goal!

A special feeling of satisfaction came over me when I was finally clear about my goals.

I realized that I wanted to reach for the stars much too hectically before, without having an exact plan. It was as if I wanted to run a marathon without thinking about equipment, training and nutrition. After I then learned how some of the most successful people of our time used these twelve steps to reach their goals, like Brian Tracy from the USA and Nikolaus B. Enkelmann from Germany, I saw myself writing down my goals with a pen in my hand and developing a plan how to reach them continuously.

I gradually studied with suffering the most successful books of the most respected coaches who were concerned with the realisation of goals. My whole way of working improved in one fell swoop and I got a better and better overview of the things I had to do.

My goal was to improve my consulting skills in the field of optical design, to triple my turnover and to get one sales deal per customer within one year.

This made me very curious about new information and insights. It was like a coincidence that I was constantly looking at the appropriate book titles. Today I am more than aware of the fact that man has a kind of unconscious filter through goal-oriented action, which sifts out exactly the information he needs in important situations in order to move forward.

So this is the reason, dear reader, why you first see these twelve important steps in front of you. Act according to these steps and you will be more and more on the road to success that you want.

CHAPTER 2

ONLY THOSE WHO KNOW THEIR GOAL CAN ACHIEVE IT

"The price for greatness is responsibility."
~ Sir Winston Churchill

Now that I had noted down my goals, I gradually began to read books about the sale. The first book was written by Frank Bettger and had the title "Lebe begeistert und gewinne!"

As a newcomer to optical consulting, I was naturally eager to find solutions with which I could better organize myself in order to increase my sales. Frank Bettger, one of the most successful salesmen of his time, helped me a lot in this respect.

In his opinion, it is of utmost importance for a salesman who wants to have success to organize his week well.1

I accepted his advice and decided on an organisation day for the week. This day fell on Sunday, when I was thinking about what I wanted to do during the week and how to best organize my time. It is therefore much more effective and relaxed to work a whole week according to a plan than to work the whole week and achieve nothing.

If you hear yourself saying now that it is nothing for me to work the whole week according to a scheme, then you must be aware that you are already acting according to a certain scheme. A scheme can be planned, but it can also be unplanned and therefore ineffective!

When I was thinking about an organized week at that time, I quickly realized how little I had planned before and how small the progress I had drawn was.

Do you sometimes not see the forest for the trees? Do you often hear yourself say that you haven't made any progress during the week? Do you often feel the urge to make faster progress?

Then take one or two hours a day a week to plan and set your goals and tasks for the week.

This will give you a better overview of your progress in the future and you will be able to gradually cut the tasks off. In addition, at the end of the week you have the good feeling that you have done everything to the best of your ability and can see yourself one step closer to your goals.

After I had completed all the tasks during the week, I was looking forward to organizing the next week and to growing with the next small and big challenges. In the further course of the book you will read how I got over two years a lot of insights into an economically strong insurance company.

There it is a basic procedure that every consultant has a weekly plan according to which he works. Get used to this secret of success and profit from it day by day.

Another good habit that many successful people have is to get up early. "Only a few people who get up late grow old. And those who are not early risers have little prospect of success in life." Benjamin Franklin recommends these two sentences to you. I have also made it my habit to get up at six o'clock every morning. So I can start the day in peace by investing an hour in reading and preparing my work. What I read in the morning is what I do on the same day.

In addition to the planned week, there is another excellent method that distinguishes a successful salesperson. Write a sales statistic! A sales statistic is a special tool to measure your sales success.

See the sales statistics as a scale. For example, if you want to lose weight, stand on the scale and immediately see how many kilos you lost during the last fitness session. That's why your sales statistics are so valuable. It shows you how much you have been able to sell by applying your newly learned skills. It is practically the measure of your progress. It was very exciting for me to follow from the very beginning how my sales per customer increased and later how the purchase turnover per customer increased.

These statistics are proof that your efforts and willingness to learn are paying off more and more. Not every employee will always be able to lend you a hand when you have concluded good deals.

But through your statistics you can recognize your achievements and reward your efforts. Therefore, make a note of your business transactions and you have your own motivation system which drives you every day. The overview will also show you immediately whether you are stagnating or even getting worse.

In this respect, you can act immediately, look at yourself and ask: "How could I have acted better? Have I asked the right questions and listened carefully? How well did I respond to the customer's wishes? In the further course of the book you will learn more about effective communication with the customer.

OPTICIAN TRAINING

A sales statistic therefore looks as follows:

week from.........to..........

Statistics of meetings and results:

Customer / Conversations / Sales / Revenues / Commission

Monday
Tuesday
Wednesday
Thursday
Friday
Saturday

Sum of the week

Difference to last week

Sum of the month to date

The writing of the sales statistics became flesh and blood for me. Every evening after work I wrote down how many customers I had talked to. I wrote down the number of sales after the meetings. Then how much the customer paid for the glasses, for example, and the provisional amount, if there was one. I might hear you say now how banal this belle may be.

Therefore, please judge it only after you have made such an overview for yourself for a long time. Then you will quickly notice how many useful formations you will gain from it, which will ultimately motivate you more.

Just the noting of the degrees made me unconsciously concentrate much more on putting a lot more ambition into the consultation and the degree. As a result, my sales turnover has increased by twenty percent after the first month!

During the day I was already looking forward to writing down in my statistics how many meetings I had in order to close a sale. All my actions were much more focused and I noticed that I was able to set very good sales targets for the day on the one hand and closing targets per customer on the other. In the beginning, there were two deals for every four customers.

Just twelve months later, I recorded a deal with almost every second customer with whom I had a meeting. You have to note that the shops of the Berlin optician mainly sold luxurious and high-quality glasses. It's amazing how writing sales statistics can improve sales management. In order to set myself an even higher goal afterwards, I concentrated on winning a deal in every conversation. This challenging goal led me to invest one hour each morning and evening per weekday in reading useful books to find out how other successful consultants achieved this goal.

In the course of this book you will read the most valuable methods for persuading your customers, which I have melted in the course of my consulting activity in ophthalmic optics. Therefore, it is best to read each chapter twice and apply the methods within the next 72 hours. Reading this book alone will not make you a successful salesman in ophthalmic optics. But if you act every day anew, then you will be surprised how quickly and effectively you will make sales.

Your customer will thank you for it. He saves time through your effective advice, comes to a decision more quickly and feels excellently taken care of by you. In the best case, he will also tell his friends about his good buying decision, which will in turn bring you new potential customers. Therefore, take full responsibility for your actions and thoughts from now on.

Consider yourself a company where you yourself are responsible for further development, time management and motivation.

Because if you do not take responsibility for yourself, then others will do it for you and steer you at will. An ugly idea, isn't it?

Have you ever heard of the 80/20 gel of Pareto? She describes that 80 percent of the results are achieved in 20 percent of the total time of a project. The remaining 20 percent of the results require 80 percent of the total time and cause the most work.

It can be applied to almost all areas of life and situations. You alone are 80 percent responsible for your success.

20 percent can be attributed to external circumstances. In companies, as well as in ophthalmic optics, 20 percent of salespeople usually account for 80 percent of turnover and thus also of commission. Do you also want to belong to the 20 percent of salespeople?

Then invest 20 percent of your time from now on with further training and exercises, which will make you an outstanding consultant in ophthalmic optics.

Because these 20 percent will create 80 percent of the value you want. You can also include your sales statistics in the next salary negotiations and draw attention to your further training in the various areas of sales. This book can be the beginning for you and provide you with very useful models that will help you achieve your goals more effectively. I still see myself today as I gathered more and more experience in these areas in the first and second year of my apprenticeship and created my own motivation.

Had I not invested 20 percent of my time and energy in studying useful books and not applied this knowledge, I would never have been able to convince customers of the value of my work and write a book about it today.

If you too adopt this model, you will quickly overcome your inner pig and motivate yourself to strive for better performance and to be better than other mediocre consultants in ophthalmic optics.

In the near future you will also encounter small and large obstacles. But you will master them if you are convinced that you want to be one of the best advisors in ophthalmic optics and act in the service of your customers. Serve the customer and he will also serve you.

In the book "The Psychology of Conviction" Robert B. Cialdini, together with other recognized professors, shows the behavior of human relationships in various studies. As an example, he noted that when we do other people a favor, you feel obliged to return the favor to us out of your reason. One may think it is a banal insight, but it is a great advantage to be aware of this behaviour when advising customers.[2]

The next time you stand in front of a client, think about it and do him a favour by giving him your best and treating him as if he were your friend.

Then he will also pay you back with a purchase for your commitment or at least recommend you to others with pleasure.

I think you may already notice what I will give you next on your way and what you would like to recommend next.

It is the emotions that play a very decisive role in advising the client. Which is the most important and why you can multiply your income and your sales success, you will read in the next chapter.

CHAPTER 3

THE PROBABLY BEST PAID QUALITY IN THE WORLD

"Honest and cordial enthusiasm is one of the most important success factors" ~ Dale Carnegie

Whenever I observe successful people today, whether they are giving a lecture in front of thousands of people or are about to sell a three million Euro house, I see again and again a very specific characteristic that distinguishes them and makes them what they are. A characteristic that awakens a certain feeling in us listeners or customers.

A Feeling of attention, tension and interest for a very specific thing. If you've ever seen a presentation by Steve Jobs about the emotion with which he sold his innovative products, you might see what I'm getting at. Just imagine how Michael Jackson fascinated his audience at the time. Listen how Barack Obama spoke to his voters for himself and how Martin Luther King delivered his famous speech "I have a dream". This way of speaking and acting will give your activity as an optician and consultant a very special polish and increase your sales turnover considerably.

It is your enthusiasm.

It was on a sunny afternoon. Since the opening in the morning, the shop has been full of restless customers who wanted to protect their eyes from the sun and meet the fashion trends of the season with new sunglasses.

As a young apprentice in my first year of apprenticeship, with little knowledge about the appearance, I saw myself standing behind the sales counter and heard myself say what I had learned about the sales activity the morning after getting up:

"To inspire others, I have to act in a spirit!"

Since I absolutely wanted to buy glasses for my customers, I decided to double my energy and enthusiasm and stand up to them as the most active and passionate consultant they have ever had. I delighted the customers with the eyewear and emphasized the fantastic benefits of the lenses they have in all sorts of sun situations.

I aroused the interest of the customers by hearing from me in which situations the glasses would serve an excellent purpose and how the wearer of the glasses would gain in comfort and style.

As a result, I myself gained more and more enthusiasm, which motivated me to advise even more actively and with even more verve.

Despite the heat and the constant customer frequency, I never got tired of getting every single customer enthusiastic about glasses again and presenting them with the desired possibilities of the products. It was simply brilliant to see how you could put a smile on the customers' faces. They were amazed at the passion and chemical enthusiasm with which a pair of glasses was presented to them.

My enthusiasm for the individual glasses was transferred to the customers within seconds. I saw how they also took on a positive mood and heard how they enjoyed their new glasses. When I came to Hause at the end of the day, I should have been completely tired. But the opposite was the case.

I myself was still full of joy about the conversations and about the customers I had made happy, so from that moment on I decided to act enthusiastically every day anew. I had never sold so many glasses in one day before and received generous praise from my store manager. Since I now also regularly wrote the sales statistics and put more and more enthusiasm into my work, my sales increased steadily.

Every new product benefit and every new insight from a eyewear company that I learned in the course of my training I enthusiastically added to the customer interview. In order to increase the variety of useful arguments that I could enthusiastically present to customers, I was interested in everything that had to do with eyeglass use and eyeglass fashion. From now on the customer should have a real desire for a certain pair of glasses.

Make your customers' glasses or product as tasty as possible When top chefs are shown at work on television, the viewer sees the chef's dedication and enthusiasm for the individual ingredients and foods that he puts in the audience's mouth. These five-star chefs have a large repertoire of knowledge about their products and share this with enthusiasm. Are you also interested in your glass types, eyeglass materials and areas of application and ignite your enthusiasm in yourself.

This enthusiasm is transferred to the customer and lets him buy it.

Say it to yourself with the words of Frank Bettger: "Handle enthusiastically and you will be inspired!"3

The decision to increase my enthusiasm helped me to absorb new information again and again and to get more knowledge about consulting in ophthalmic optics.

Take the decision to put more enthusiasm into your advice. Spirituality lets you overcome your nervousness and transforms it into activity. In addition, your activity and enthusiasm will infect your employees and colleagues and they will soon act as you do. Have you ever listened to a lecture where you almost fell asleep? Do you still see the bored salesman in front of you asking for a different trouser size? Then you now also know how important this chapter is for you if you want to fascinate your customers with your glasses.

In the next chapter you will learn how to increase not only your enthusiasm, but also your sympathy and attraction to your customers.

CHAPTER 4

HOW TO CREATE SYMPATHY TO THE CUSTOMER THROUGH MIRRORING

"If you want to convince a person of something, you must first convince them that you are their sincere friend."
~ *Abraham Lincoln*

Why is it so important for you to create sympathy for your customer? Surely you can remember a situation in your life in which you were in complete harmony with another person. Recall these experiences for yourself once more in your thoughts. Look at the posture of your conversation partner and compare it with yours.

Listen once again to the choice of words you use to describe your counterpart. Did you often choose the same words? Did you both speak in colloquial language, or rather formally?

Have your voices adjusted in pitch, speed and rhythm?

Were you in agreement with the other person about the content of the conversation and therefore your mood was similar?

If you agree to this now, then you probably felt a high degree of sympathy for your conversation partner. You were familiar with each other.

This is a natural phenomenon and in this day and age an important insight in order to establish a sympathetic relationship with complete strangers in a relatively short time. If a politician, TV presenter or mother wants to build up a good relationship with a person, then you have to create a friendly and sympathetic atmosphere.

Exactly this is done by the law of similarity.

Whether you meet a person with the same haircut or a person from the same football club, or a person with a similar attitude to you.

With similarities, you can get to a common wire more quickly and at best have an excellent time.

What good will it do you if your customer finds you immediately likeable?

You want to be useful to your customer and sell him good products? Then convince him that he feels friendly with you and that he finds you sympathetic! When I first heard about this kind of communication in a sales seminar, I was overwhelmed by the numerous unconscious processes that take place during a conversation with other people.

During this time I gained a lot of knowledge about this approach and applied it continuously in the consultations.

On the following days I immediately applied this knowledge and the results were simply fantastic!

Imagine completely resetting your ego and fully adjusting to the other person through body language, voice and word choice.

First of all, your customer will feel familiar with you very quickly because he will feel your well-being.

Secondly, you will be surprised how gladly your customer will open up to you and entrust you with his concerns and wishes.

And thirdly, the customer is much more open to your suggestions and your advice will be accepted.

You can have a lot of fun selling if you train this method and use it again and again until it becomes a part of your character. As a side-effect, you will make a satisfied smile on the customer's face and get more sales.

How do you immediately create sympathy with your customers?

Mirror the body postures and movements of your customers inconspicuously. That is, you take something time-delayed similar attitudes or movements.

For example, your customer puts his left hand in his left trouser pocket, then you put your right hand in your trouser pocket with a slight delay.

If your customer adopts a stable body posture with his chest outstretched, then you also adopt your posture without appearing ridiculous.

It is only a matter here of resembling the attitude of the customer, so that he unconsciously perceives you as equal or equal.

Then equal your voice to that of your counterpart. If your customer speaks in a very deep voice, then you also speak rather deeply.

If your customer tells you slowly and calmly about his needs, then ask him also slowly and calmly further. If he softly tells you about his visual ailments, then talk softly about the causes.

Then mirror your favourite words or expressions. I once mirrored a customer who made me understand how difficult it had been for him to buy a bril-driver and simply nothing good was available for him to choose from. His appearance was very casual and relaxed.

At first glance, it didn't seem to be like our typical customers, who often came to our store in business attire and formal manner. In addition, he used a very casual colloquial language and tended to be authoritarian due to his low vocal pitch and very precise manner of expression. In short, he asked me to give him the perfect glasses. So I adjusted my behaviour to his and asked him what he would like most about his future wish glasses?

In his colloquial language he told me how much he liked glasses with "fat emblems" on the temples.

I then presented him with a pair of glasses, which applied, and in the same words I emphasized the "fat emblems" on the sides. I often asked him questions such as: "How long have you been looking for glasses?" or: "On what special occasions would you wear sunglasses?

The more answers he gave me, the better I could reflect his body language and idioms.

The customer promptly felt at one level with me and only when looking at the price did he realize that the "fat emblems" on the sides were real sterling silver. He had never seen sunglasses for 1,750 euros before. I mirrored him further and took over even more his choice of words.

After all, we were so familiar with each other that we both enjoyed our conversation and the customer decided to buy the glasses.

It is quite conceivable that other opticians did not feel like adjusting to him in order to create a familiar relationship. In the worst case, they might have looked down on him from above. The fact is, the customer apparently felt understood for the first time in our conversation and was thus delighted by glasses.

In the end, this customer was even able to treat himself to "high-end" glasses! So if you want to be one of those opticians who can successfully sell to even the most difficult or complicated customers, then take this approach and your next big success will come very soon.

In the next step, in addition to the sympathy of the manufacturer, it is important to address the right buying motives with your customers.

CHAPTER 5

RECOGNIZE TYPES OF BUYERS

"Whoever does what he already can always remains what he already is." ~ Henry Ford

In order for you as an optician to better understand the needs of your customers, it is important to know how the motif and emotion system is designed in the customer's mind.

The motif systems explain to us which glasses the customer buys and why. Together with the Nymphenburg Group, Dr. Hans Georg Häusel has conducted research to better understand consumers and has developed a scientifically based motif system for sales practice:

1. the balance system
2. the stimulant system and
3. the dominance system

What's the point of knowing these buyer types?

Please think again about this. Back to an experience with a seller who wanted to sell you something, but tried to "convince" you with the wrong topics. For example, you want to chew a car and the seller tells you about the "thick rims" or the "high horsepower number".

Didn't you quickly get bored of these uninteresting topics and start to see escape actions in you, although you actually wanted to buy a "very safe, reliable and fuel-efficient" car?

Well, even mediocre to inexperienced opticians make this mistake by not recognizing the buyer type of the customer and addressing the wrong/uninteresting topics.

You win the customer over faster as an optician and achieve sales more easily if you address the most important and interesting topics for the customer that satisfy his buying motives!

The buying motives are different depending on the type of buyer. We therefore differentiate between three central buyer types:

1. The dominance type:

He wants power, status and superiority. He wants to assert himself, strive upwards and be better than everyone else.

He is very active and wants to increase his power. Performance counts for him!

His buying motive is particularly noticeable in status products, such as expensive watches, fashion, VIP status, expensive cars, exquisite wines, products and services that speak strength and speed, fitness products, products and services that increase his performance.

If we meet customers who have such an appearance and show the characteristics described above, we can classify them as dominant types.

How can you best sell to the dominant types?

You can sell a dominant type especially rare glasses, for example made of gold, natural horn or wood, because he can satisfy his exquisite taste and his connoisseurship before friends, acquaintances and family members.

You can also sell him glasses that are particularly popular with people and at best are worn by celebrities in Hollywood movies or musicians. For example, Ray Ban Aviator pilot glasses will be worn by former heads of state such as Barack Obama or Nicolas Sarkozy, but also by actor Tom Cruise and others.

This customer also likes to be inspired by prestigious and expensive brand glasses such as Boss, Prada or Chrome Hearts. He therefore also likes brand logos that represent his status. I count Robert Geiss among these dominant types, for example.

He is enthusiastic about the latest fashion glasses that can be found in the current issues of GQ or other men's magazines.

For this person, very good looks are also of central importance and everything that favours them makes his heart beat faster.

They therefore score with him with glasses that suit him particularly well and emphasize his attractiveness. In the chapter on colour and type advice, you will also learn everything you need to know.

2. The stimulant type:

This customer wants experience, something new and individual. He is looking for new adventures or experiences, wants to break away from the familiar, avoid boredom and be as attractive as possible.

The consumer likes to try out new products, trends and innovations. The consumer's buying motive is particularly visible: in consumer electronics, the travel industry, experience gastronomy, all kinds of nutritious products, products that help him to be different from everyone else, innovative products in terms of design, experience shopping, music, videos, information via newsletters and invitations to events.

If we recognize the above characteristics at the customer, we can easily classify this as a stimulant type.

How can you sell to the stimulant type?

This type loves to buy glasses that have elaborate colors and shapes that you rarely see. He is often dressed in colour and his glasses are supposed to underline the style. These customers love special features of the glasses, such as certain patterns or temple systems for changing. Also this customer likes complex processing at eyeglasses and individual materials such as wood or special plastics, which exhibit special characteristics, such as ease or flexibility.

These customers are also enthusiastic about special glass properties such as photochromic or polarization.

Stimulant types also have an eye for beautiful spectacle shapes for their face and pay great attention to them.

How to quickly select the right shapes and colours is explained in the lesson on colour and type advice.

New eyewear brands can also help you win over this type of customer, as they like to discover and try out new things. Therefore, always show the so-called eyewear novelties and trends first!

Stimulation customers love eye-catching glasses. So, as a professional, quench your thirst for this purchase motive!

Put together a selection of eyeglasses that let the customer stand out in the grey mass of uniformity through individuality and conspicuousness.

3. The balance type:

This customer most wants the motif security. He strives for peace and harmony.

He prefers to avoid every danger, every change, is a habitual person and likes to avoid insecurity.

His buying motive is particularly visible in all types of insurance, e.g. pension schemes, security measures, reliable quality, long product life, guarantees, reliable service, advice, traditional products that have been known for a long time, the same contact person, family businesses, personal customer relations.

A customer with these safety-related features is immediately recognized as a Balance Type.

How can you best sell to the Balance type now?

As mentioned earlier, the Balance Type loves security. So you score with it with glasses that have a high UV protection and a glass material that is as unbreakable as possible.

An equally important purchase criterion for him is good and reliable vision with glasses.

Examples of this motif are certain lens shades or a super spectacle that offers the highest level of satisfaction for the specified lenses. You can also tell these customers about the stable and shatterproof eyewear material.

For example, emphasize the shatterproof properties of stainless steel or titanium or advocate the shatterproof plastic lenses, which in the event of an accident do not shatter like glass into single parts.

Many spectacles also have durable materials (titanium, stainless steel) that require little care. Or special acetate plastics, whose "plasticizers" remain in the material longer and thus guarantee long-lasting comfort.

The lightness of a pair of glasses is also important to him if it sits particularly gently on the nose and provides long-lasting comfort.

Last but not least, you can also convince this customer with services if you emphasise and offer them. Regular spectacle adjustments, eye checks or guarantee promises for certain lenses or spectacles have made the heart of this customer beat particularly high. This type of customer also likes it when you establish a personal relationship with him and take time for his needs. As a thank you, this type of customer will remain loyal to you because they are interested in long-term relationships.

Now that you can discover and address the right buying motives for your respective customers, let us also look at the customer's sensory channels to be convinced.

CHAPTER 6

NLP - CONVINCING IN THE LANGUAGE OF THE CUSTOMER

"Every action is preceded by a thought!"
~ Ralph Waldo Emerson

Why should you now speak in the customer's language in order to be able to sell more?

Basically, each of us has the feeling of selling. Why do I say that?

Well, please take a look back at the time when you were really in love with a person.

Remember the first days you got together fresh. Can you still see in your mind's eye what you have done to show people how much they have meant to you?

What did you tell him, what did you show him and how did you touch him?

We know these situations either from ourselves or have already taken them into account once in other couples in love.

As an example:

You see a couple sitting on a park bench, freshly in love, and notice how the young man, Philip, signals his affection to his lover, Lisa.

He sits facing her and kisses her cheeks. He holds her hand and expresses his feelings to her in the liveliest words. He also shows her a little present next.

So, what's young Philip doing there? That's right. He tries to show himself from his best side and to sell Lisa by all means he knows. And that, dear reader, is exactly what this lesson is all about.

The young man in love uses the most effective means to be on the same wavelength with the people he meets.

So what exactly is used here and what are the benefits for you in terms of sales?

It is the NLP (Neurolinguistic Programming) that Philip unknowingly uses. NLP is a method developed by psychologists to put patients into a desired positive state faster and more effectively.

This method is already widely used today and is increasingly being taught in management, team and sales training.

Therefore it is particularly valuable for you as an optician working in sales to use this method.

According to NLP we find that every person has three sensory channels with which he can communicate:

1. the visual channel
2. the auditory channel
3. the kinesthetic channel

So that Philip can now convince his lover of himself, he uses all three channels to show her how much he likes her.

"He sits facing her and kisses her cheeks. Here he uses his tactile sense (kinesthetic).

"...expresses his feelings in the liveliest words". He lets Lisa hear what she means to him (auditory).

"He also shows her a little present next." He presents her something to mo- tive her over her sight (visually).

Philip certainly reaches his goal with the method of addressing all three sensory channels.

But: People always have a sense channel, which they prefer the most!

After all, what happens now when the once fresh lovers have already been together for a year? As an example: Lisa (kinesthetically inclined) will complain to Philip (visually inclined) because she doesn't get as many touches and kisses from Philip as she did at the beginning of her time on the park bench. So if Philip is clever now, he recognizes Lisa's preferred sensory channel and can make her happy again and again.

So that you can be on the same wavelength with your customer as quickly as possible, you have to find out which sensory channel the customer prefers. It is not important to be 100 percent right. Some people also use two sensory channels almost equally.

What is the point of speaking in the customer's language?

The methods described in this lesson are intended to give you a better understanding of your customers, so that you can be 80 percent right with your assessment in order to successfully discuss and advise them according to their sensory channels.

When I put glasses on the counter of a customer of mine, we call her Mrs. Weiß, in front of her eyes, she said the following:

"Wow, look at these colors! I've always wanted to see exactly this mixture of colours on myself.

How did they make the brown shades shine like that? This kind of brown tone is very rare! Also, the shape of the glasses looks good. I have to see how it looks on me." That's how she described her thoughts. This example shows very clearly that Mrs. Weiß thinks and speaks through the visual senses.

In order to make them even more aware of the glasses, I chose a very descriptive language and emphasized the visual characteristics of the glasses even more:

"Imagine, the glasses are processed with a high-quality plastic, so that this unique color mixture originates from it. Look, the manufacturer polishes the glasses three times to make them shine so fantastically. You can see that the designer orientates himself in colours and shapes according to the latest fashion trends. Take another look in the mirror to see the effect with the glasses!

As you can see now, I used words like: see, imagine, know, take a look.

Thus I achieved two effects with my customer:

1. she felt understood, because I concentrated on her language and thus on her sensory perception.

2. their emotions were strengthened by my descriptive language and I could inspire them even more.

The customer bought the glasses within ten minutes! She didn't need longer to decide, because I emphasized the visual qualities of the glasses once again for her, so that she could convince herself of the desired advantages.

That's all!

Very often it happens that I look at a T-shirt in a shop and think to myself: "Lucky hit, a super cut", whereupon a salesman comes closer and presents me three other T-shirts in addition, instead of simply asking myself whether I like exactly this T-shirt. Had he done it, he could have saved himself and me time. Here he would drive what exactly I like about the T-shirt, so that the seller can deal with these details more strongly with his communication.

Therefore, dear reader, consider that successful consultants switch off their ego and concentrate exactly on what the customer really wants and package it in the language of the customer and not in their own!

For this reason, I consider the well-known proverb: "Treat people the way you want to be treated yourself" to be insufficient for sales. Why?

For example, a customer who mostly perceives a product kinesthetically, who likes to feel a product in order to feel its value. If a consultant now thinks (visually) that he has to serve the customer according to his own sensory channel and show him other details, then it is difficult or impossible for him to conclude.

In the previous chapter of this book you will learn how to deal with different types of buyers. Here you will see why the proverb mentioned above can be regarded as outdated in sales with these presented methods.

How can you now speak in the customer's language?

As previously discussed, people mainly think in three different sensory channels:

The first sensory channel is the visual one, which concentrates on colours, shapes and sizes. This is most common in people.

The second sensory channel is the auditory one, so that volume and key play an important role. This is the second most common channel in humans.

The third most common sensory channel is the ki- nesthetic one. This channel is about the condition of an object as well as its weight and feeling.

It can also happen, as described, that two sensory channels are equally present and perceived in humans.

A customer who uses a very visual language and is therefore mainly motivated via the visual channel is best recognized and convinced by the following visual words: see, recognize, show and crystal clear.

For example, you can mention: "Please look at these warm colors of the glasses. You will soon know how harmoniously they match your skin tone."

A customer who uses a very auditory language and is therefore mainly motivated via the auditory channel is most likely to be identified and persuaded with the following auditory words:

hear, sound, harmonize, sound, tune in.

For example, you can ask: "Do you like to be tuned in by modern or more classical glasses? What would we hear from your husband about these glasses?

You will discover and convince a customer who uses a very kinaesthetic language and is therefore mainly motivated via the kinaesthetic channel with the following kinaesthetic words: feel, touch, hard, soft, firm, immobile. For example, you can say: "You like to touch this material once in a while. It is firm and stable. This makes many people who wear glasses feel safe."

You will quickly see how effective and easy it will be to motivate your customers to buy glasses more quickly. The more often you practice these things, the more secure you will feel and the more grateful customer voices you will hear.

CHAPTER 7

BENEFIT-INSTEAD CHARACTERISTIC REASONING

"You have to lure the fish with a bait he likes."
~ *Dale Carnegie*

Why is benefit instead of feature argumentation important? In principle, many opticians make the mistake of speaking only of the features of the lenses in order to convince the customer. They then talk about super reflections, polarizations, refractive indices and so on.

The problem is that no customer buys pure features!

Features = Properties of products or services.

The refractive index of 1.6 is a glass characteristic. The stainless steel flexibility of a spectacle frame is a material feature.

But what the customer buys in the end are the advantages he has when using the product!

Benefits = advantages of products or services that arise for the customer in daily life.

For example, the customer wants to look good with glasses, be dazzled little by the sun, have glasses for several purposes or glasses that his child will not break.

What does the benefit-instead-characteristic argumentation bring to you?

Customers always think about what is important to them and where a product or service can help them.

That's why professional opticians never argue pure features of lenses or spectacle frames professionals always emphasize the benefits or advantages a customer has with the use of glasses, because customers can better understand them! It is not your job as an optician to train the customer to become an optician yourself or to bore him with details, but to give him important advantages. At the same time, as opticians they know how to put themselves in the position and ideas of the customer, because they are forced to talk about the advantages for the customer and not to annoy the customer with their own opinions or personal advantages. The customer feels thereby immediately understood by them.

When it comes to new things, people have only a limited capacity to absorb new information.

By the predominant use Argu mentationen you make sure that the customer gets all important information in shortest time, which motivates him to the purchase of eyeglasses. As a professional, you make a faster conclusion!

How do you implement the benefit-instead-feature argumentation?

Since your goal is to close the sale, please make a note of a number of reasons, i.e. advantages, why your customer should buy each lens design or eyeglass material. Please choose the three most important advantages! Then you can use a brief justification of the benefit by means of a feature.

Example: Stainless steel spectacle frame Advantages

1. "Your child cannot accidentally break or injure your glasses while playing due to the flexibility and therefore stability of the material".

2. "You don't have painful bruises on your nose like other heavier materials because of the lightness of the material."

3. "You can wear this frame forever and save money due to the rust resistance and the longevity of the material, which is superior to plastic."

Example: Polarization lenses Advantages

1. "They are far superior to other anglers when it comes to fishing and can place their baits better because they can see the fish under the surface of the water, because these glasses eliminate the reflections of the sun's water".

2. "You get a glare-free and razor-sharp view when skiing and you are even safer on the way, because these glasses reduce the reflections as well as the shine of the snow surface to over 90%.

3. "You have a more relaxed view when sailing your boat, you don't need to pinch your eyes when the sun is strong and you can stand it longer in the sun because these lenses remove over 90% of the strong light reflections from the water surface.

This is why it is so important to ask the customer questions in advance, such as: "In which situations do you need sunglasses particularly frequently?" or "Which wishes should glasses fulfil for you? As a professional, you can fulfil the wishes that customers have for glasses by highlighting the advantages of glasses or lenses that match the wishes of the customers. It is simple and yet 80% of opticians do not implement it. In your argumentation, as you may have already noticed, you always proceed as follows:

(What is the benefit for the customer? Advantage:)

"They no longer have painful pressure points on their noses because..."

(Now give the simple/short reason:)

"... because the stainless steel material is much lighter than conventional plastic glasses!"

In this way you can give the customer three of the most important advantages for him! In this way, you ensure that the customer remembers them and that they are mentally unhooked. This makes it much easier for you to sell your eyeglasses, more user-friendly and, above all, faster!

If you have already internalized the three types in the Buyers Types lesson, then you can add an "and" to the argumentation. In this way you can specifically address the motivation of the customer on the basis of his buyer type.

An example of this:

"You no longer have any painful pressure points on your nose, because the stainless steel material is many times lighter than that of the plastic glasses and you therefore feel more comfort in the long term." (here: a balance type with the safety motif)

Or in the type of adventure that new it / individual motivates, you add that it "...and in addition carries a very individual material."

In addition, you can mention the performer type, who is interested in performance and consideration, who thus possesses one of the most powerful materials, which is produced by German engineering.

In addition to the types of buyers, we can also distinguish between sales to men and women, about which you will learn more in the next chapter.

CHAPTER 8

WOMEN BUY DIFFERENTLY FROM MEN

"Do you know many languages ~ do you have many keys for a lock?"- -Voltaire

Why should you always be divided between women and men in counselling and sales in ophthalmic optics?

Women account for over 70 % of disposable income. Therefore opticians finally have to take off their unisex glasses in order to reach men and women! Because, women decide to over 70% on the purchase of consumer goods. That describes among other things the brain researcher Hans George Husel in its book Brain Script and deals there still with important purchase differences, to which we come back later!

You have probably already noticed that the majority of your customers are women in ophthalmic optics. If you want to understand why women tick or shop differently from men, you first have to realize that women's consciousness is influenced by their hormone estrogen. It is responsible for women's softness and tolerance. It also has an effect on her open and positive emotional state.

Men, on the other hand, are controlled by the hormone testosterone. It causes a simple and euphoric thinking in men, so that men like to simplify and systematize things. In addition, this hormone drives men and promotes dominance thinking.

Women, on the other hand, have a highly developed imagination because their right brain half is more activated. Men, on the other hand, are more likely to use their logical thinking because their left brain hemisphere is more stimulated.

What good does it do you now to address and advise women differently from men?

It is important for women to increase their attractiveness in order to have as good an effect as possible on a man of their choice. Thus, women rather buy from design and beauty motifs. It is therefore crucial for opticians to address such product characteristics in women in order to achieve faster and more frequent sales.

Since women are very caring, they also buy gifts five times more often than men and therefore form a powerful buying target group for opticians. Safety is also very important to them. As a result, women are more likely to opt for glasses if they are advised on the subject of safety and reliability. Men, on the other hand, love products that give them power and are predictable.

Thus, sales-boosting opticians also know how to align product descriptions to these motifs in order to convince more quickly. Brands such as Hugo Boss, for example, already carry these motifs within themselves. Technical gimmicks also make men's hearts beat faster, especially when they can still create a feeling of superiority. Glasses made of special materials, such as wood or stainless steel, for example, which are also rare to buy, can score highly with men!

Men should therefore first demonstrate the technical refinements of the glasses and try them out on their own. Instead, women should first and foremost recognise the design and reliability of the glasses and also have to face them.

This information alone will make you an above-average consultant in the eyes of your customers, because you will understand and serve their needs much faster.

What is the best way to convince women?

Basically, women motivate product descriptions with rather soft words that produce a soft sound. For example, "...the soft material gives the glasses a very supple fit" or "This frame with its soft colours is very harmless to your hair".

Or "...Michael Kors glasses offer you an elegant and well thought-out design language".

You can also say the following: "Feel once how smooth and dazzling this valuable plastic is polished."

Since safety and reliability are important purchasing motives for women, describe to the customer how reliable a certain spectacle frame can be in the event of an accident, or how safe a plastic lens is for children compared to mineral lenses.

UV protection filters or other glass tints also provide a very convincing safety motif for women.

Simplicity in handling glasses or contact lenses is just as important for women as the quality of materials.

Materials, for example, can be soft to wear and feel particularly smooth or appear very valuable due to their shine or colour mixture.

Women also like it very much to stimulate their imagination, since their right brain half is strongly active through the estrogen and provides for creative thinking.

Therefore, decorate grateful situations for the women:

For example, you can describe a picture of a customer sitting at a café on a sunny day in Rome.

Here she can now relax and read a newspaper through the colour gradient glass, as the lower half of the glass is brighter and protects the upper half from the dazzling afternoon sun.

Try to ask a lot of information in which the customer uses the glasses and convince her with thought games.

Because women are more social beings than men and have more of a sense of togetherness, it is also important for them to be able to confirm their environment.

They have certainly often observed that women usually go shopping accompanied or seek the advice of their girlfriend or partner. Here it is particularly important to include the companion when buying glasses in the conversation, as they can often even have the last word.

So when women come in company, it is professional if you sell yourself and your advice not only to the customer but also to everyone else. Because the customer will ask her companion for her opinion and if she is not convinced, the customer will doubt and not buy. As an ex- perte in the consultation with all clients, you should therefore have as balanced a proportion as possible and proactively include the accompaniment:

For example, you may ask the escort how much the customer likes the frame and fit of a pair of glasses.

Remember positive remarks and mention them in changed form during the course of the conversation to encourage the customer in her choice.

Negative statements by the escort about glasses are immediately recorded and passed on to the customer as a question in order to find out whether the customer thinks similarly.

Thus, opinions can either be continued, e.g. through the presentation of alternative glasses, or invalidated if the customer has a different point of view. This may be the case if, for example, she has different ideas about glasses than her companions. Her goal is to also function as a moderator in this consultation and thus to keep the sales conversation with many questions on the go.

You lead your customer and their companions to a purchase decision with which everyone is happy at best.

Furthermore, according to scientific research, women have a distinct sense of balance, which makes values such as satisfaction and service important to them. Therefore, please discuss the satisfaction guarantees of the glasses or frames and offer services.

This can include polishing of the frames or regular checks of the brilliance.

Think about services that you would like to offer free of charge, whereby you can name many here!

With it you take the customer her vision, since she feels well taken care of by your service with you.

How can you win men over quickly and easily to buy glasses?

Men are much more enthusiastic about technical product features than women. Therefore, show them how flexible the stainless steel material can be bent and how superior it is to other glasses due to its lightness. Demonstrate the function of polarizing lenses and show how they can look through the surface of the playing water to recognize lenses or eliminate polarization reflections in the snow. Always emphasize the sophisticated and exciting product features and advantages of the glasses!

Men also like it when you, as a sales expert, give them orientation through the variety of glasses in your shop.

If you have asked the customer what shapes and colours he wants, then let him know that certain eyeglass shelves in your shop and certain brands or frames are out of the question.

This makes it easier for him to make his decision, because he prefers orderly and simple thinking.

He feels understood by you and accepts you immediately as an expert, because you relieve him in the decision making. You have to describe to him which shapes and colours are best suited for him and which strongly limit him.

Men may also have more square and straight forms, but with them they appear masculine and strong.

Therefore, you should rather choose these forms first in order to convince the customer more quickly.

What men are just as enthusiastic about is recognition and status. They want recognition from women, family and friends. If glasses can give them this feeling, then they buy them.

You can create recognition by asking a female companion or colleague for their opinion on the glasses. You can also mention how quickly the customer can demonstrate the technical gimmicks of his glasses to his relatives and colleagues.

You give them status when their glasses are worn by celebrities, for example, or appear in movies.

Fashion brands are also proof of status, as are the precious metals gold or sterling silver on glasses.

Men are more convinced of such things than most opticians would expect.

I have sold significantly more price-intensive gold, silver, wood or natural horn brils to men than to women. Show such unique glasses to men and you will see!

Male customers activate you with do- minanten product descriptions.

For example, the frame is enormously strong and unbreakable due to the titanium material, as this is far superior to others. Or, a certain frame made of stainless steel is German engineering art, since it can be opened independently without screws, so that the customer can change the sunglasses if necessary and remains calculable for him every sun situation. You can also tell him with a smile that according to an article in GQ Magazine, for example, most men find the shape of the glasses you recommend most attractive to women.

It also makes sense to describe a particular eyewear brand with brands from outside the industry, for example by mentioning: "This brand is considered the Porsche of eyewear".

You now know the differences that motivate men and women to buy a pair of glasses. A method that will make it easier for both of them to make a purchase decision will be learnt in the next chapter.

CHAPTER 9

THE 3-GLASSES-RULE

"Life offers so much more possibilities when you realize that everything around us was created by people who weren't smarter than you." ~ Steve Jobs

Why should you actually apply a certain 3-glasses-rule?

Please put yourself in the following frame of mind: You are standing in a grocery store in front of a reunion with jam and would like to buy a strawberry jam. To your amazement, the retailer means "particularly good" and presents eleven different varieties of strawberry jam. What is your first thought? Do you feel overwhelmed?

In the worst case, with the variety of choices available, you will no longer be interested in breaking your head over a strawberry arm drawer, save yourself the trouble and reach for the nearest Nutella glass.

How can this thought game be transferred to sales in ophthalmic optics?

Well, in the last ten years, when I have visited different opticians out of interest in order to let their concepts and advice have an effect on me, I have noticed one thing again and again: The advising opticians always meant it particularly well with their customers and put an abundance of glasses in front of them to demonstrate their "variety".

The customer, overburdened by the oversupply of different spectacle shapes and colours, was usually quickly demotivated.

Like many other customers, he usually understands very little about glasses and can therefore distinguish them even less from each other.

To the disadvantage of the optician! Because the customer feels an uncertainty of decision in those moments. Too much choice blocks his view of the essential things. It should be essential for the customer that he only sees glasses within his grasp, which he puts on the short list through a conscious exclusion process.

The professional exclusion procedure is known to the opticians with the highest sales and is used specifically to lead their customers quickly and easily to a purchase decision. So far, so good.

So how does the 3 glasses rule work?

The principle is as follows. Only a maximum of three glasses are ever placed within reach of the customer!

These glasses have their place only serves, because they were selected in advance by the optician through targeted needs assessment and assessment of the fit on the customer.

If a pair of glasses does not fit properly, if the colour does not look good or if it has a flaw expressed by the customer, it is immediately excluded and sorted out.

What the customer ultimately sees in front of him is a "selection" of the glasses that are most useful and suitable for him.

And now the decisive thing about this method is what follows.

With three choices, people usually opt for the "middle second choice". Even the psychologist Robert B. Cialdini confirmed this phenomenon in his book "Die Psychologie des überzeugenens" (The Psychology of Conviction).

For example, if you ask a Starbucks salesperson which coffee size is sold the most, they will answer "the middle one". Try it out for yourself!

The professional optician presents the customer with three glasses on the table. In the middle he places the glasses, which he considers to be optimal for the customer, a deliberately cheaper and less attractive pair of glasses on the left position. And in the right position he places the most expensive glasses, which, however, also meet the customer's taste very well.

As an optician, what good is the 3-glasses-rule for you now?

The customer will be motivated by the limited choice and the simple overview to decide to buy. The professional eye optician, however, also limits the options.

In 80% of the cases, the customer will opt for the "golden mean" and shop with a good feeling of self-determination. In 20% of the cases, the customer will even opt for the expensive third pair of glasses and earn the optician a higher turnover.

As an optician, you make the customer's two favourites more attractive with this method and simply make the decision easier for him.

So please learn from my own practice as an optician and apply this tried and tested method to every customer. Your increase in sales and your sales figures will confirm this!

CHAPTER 10

FIRST GIVE, THEN TAKE

"Pay any debt, as if God were writing the bill."
~ Ralph Waldo Emerson

Why should you give first in the sales process, before you take?

Remember a last visit to a restaurant, where the friendly waiter not only brought the bill to your table, but also served you a small candy or a schnapps at home.

Did you enjoy this little surprise? What was going on in you?

Did you then give this waiter a more generous tip than other waiters who didn't give you a little present?

Or remember a friend who once invited you to his birthday. Didn't that motivate you to invite him to your next party?

If you agree with these thought games, then you unconsciously follow the reciprocity rule. Simply put, we rather give something back to a person if we have received something from them in advance. If I give you something for your birthday, you would like to return the favor and also give me a present.

We would like to vanch ourselves for favors, in order not to appear as stingy or ungrateful.

This behavior takes place partly unconsciously in us humans, since we are conditioned as social humans.

The professor of psychology, Robert B. Cialdini, had already carried out an ex-periment years ago to uncover the power of this rule. He found out that a stranger finds someone rather likeable if they do her a favour or give her a small present. In addition, the donated persons are also much more willing to do the giver a favor, for example to chew lots from him.10

Even an old proverb says that giving is more blessed than taking!

Especially when we meet foreign customers for the first time, it is of utmost importance to first establish a friendly and friendly relationship with the person.

What is the point of giving first?

You have an enormous effect on your customers through the principle of giving.

First of all your customer will find you more sympathetic, because he feels your goodwill towards him.

Of course, it is a prerequisite that you implement this principle out of deepest feeling and benevolence towards the customer. Not every customer will buy expensive varifocals from you, but you will sprinkle the seed, which will flourish later, in the form of a purchase or a recommendation.

Because the customer will be grateful to you and in the best case will want to return the favor immediately. Either it motivates him more to buy glasses from you, or it stimulates him to buy more than he actually intended. I often achieved astonishingly high sales with just one customer. I like to remember a sales talk with a new customer, who ordered a pair of varifocals, sunglasses with corrective lenses and reading glasses from me because of this approach.

The turnover on this day in 2009 was over 2.000 € with only one customer.

If you have put a lot of effort in the run-up to the event, regarding the pleasure or the gift, your customer will perceive this unconsciously. How high will the value or benefit of a paid service be - but much higher!

What is the best way to apply this rule?

As an optician, you can apply this rule very easily and quickly because you are always in close contact with your customer.

So do the following. If you greet the customer and he gives you his glasses, for example, then proactively suggest that you clean them briefly or polish them with a cloth. You can also tighten and check the screws at the same time.

When you have finished, for example, give him a free cleaning cloth in his hand. In addition, many opticians have custom-made cleaning cloths with their logos on them, so they also give the customer advertising in their business. So you have already done him three favours and immediately make him happier!

If you then carry out the authorization analysis with the customer and he tells you about his wishes, you can say the following:

"I think I understand which wishes your new glasses should fulfil and will pick out a small collection for you right away. Would you like some water, coffee or tea?" Your customer answers: "With pleasure!

Then serve your customers the coffee they want on a nice saucer with spoon, sugar or milk jug and place a lot of value on the arrangement of the whole thing, as if it were in a five-star hotel.

You can also add a little candy or something similar to coffee to your customer's coffee as a "little shopping boost".

I can guess what you're thinking now. So much effort? So much value on little things and details? And any extra sweets to go with it?

Yes, just as much or more! Surprise your customers! Place just as much value on the preparatory work as on the advice. Your customer will unconsciously appreciate your commitment and see your further advice as higher quality if you put a lot of love into details.

You can also surprise them with great things, such as homemade smoothies in summer or hot chocolate in winter. Be creative and stand out from the crowd to stay in the customer's memory.

Now come to the fourth courtesy.

Give the customer an extremely generous and competent consultation, which contains all aspects of this video training. For example, give the customer well-fitting glasses with perfect colour for his skin type and base your choice on the knowledge that you receive, for example, from the lesson on colour and type advice.

Very few opticians have this knowledge or apply it correctly. This means that you clearly distinguish yourself from other opticians in the eyes of your customer and do your customer a favour, because he will finally receive competent advice and can rely completely on your professionalism.

Furthermore, you can proactively offer him gifts in the form of services at the end of the sales talk. You can choose between free home delivery of the glasses or small discounts for the purchase of two glasses at the same time.

It is also a good idea to donate a case for his previous glasses if he decides to buy a new one. It is also a good idea to offer your customers small snacks on Fridays or Saturdays, "as a refreshment for long shopping days". You may invest in small things in advance, but your sales or your provisions will be able to dwindle!

This rule has an enormous effect, dear reader. So please use it wisely and give something out of the joy of giving. Then it will be given back to you with the same joy.

In the next chapter you will learn something about a very special favor that you can offer your customers.

CHAPTER 11
COLOR - AND TYPE CONSULTING

"You never get a second chance to make a first impression"
~ Will Rogers

Why should you as an optician know your way around colour and type consulting?

In my opinion, colour and type consultation should be a fundamental part of ophthalmic training, as it contributes far more to the success of the consultation than being able to draw endless beam lengths of prescription lenses. In the end, the only thing that matters in ophthalmic practice is to "conceal" the right spectacles to the customer precisely, with which he not only sees very well, but also looks very good!

The colour and type consultation therefore makes it possible to classify customers into one of four colour types and thus recommend the matching colours to their skin and hair colours.

Since my parents run hairdressing and beauty companies, I already acquired this knowledge in the second year of my optician training with their help about colour and type consultation by them.

After this knowledge has become flesh and blood through consistent practice and observation, my turnover and sales of glasses have increased further!

My customers were amazed when they found out from me which colour type they were and why they should wear a certain colour! It increased my competence so much that I was on my way to become one of the strongest sales opticians in the company with four branches at that time. During the training!

Every employee was able to track this at any time through the internal statistics of eyeglass sales.

Dear reader, I am not writing you this because I would like to state, but because you should guess how successful you can make this knowledge! This knowledge can make you one of the 20% of opticians in the company who generate 80% of the turnover and earn the most with it!

So let's get started.

Basically, this apprenticeship divides people into either warm or cold skin types based on their skin and hair colour. There are two categories of warm skin types, which are often referred to as spring or autumn. For cold skin types there are also two categories, which are often classified as summer or winter.

The theory of origin is based on Ca- role Jackson's book "Color me beautiful", to which I refer here.

What does colour and type consulting in eyewear sales bring you now?

Through colour and type advice, you can first of all immediately divide the customer into a cold or warm skin type and exclude colours in your mind that will not suit the customer well at all.

Secondly, you can limit the customer to exactly those colours that will suit him best.

Thirdly, you immediately save time, as you immediately select only the glasses that match the customer's colour type.

Fourthly, your customer will be delighted because he will look good with your choice of colour and will consider you to be competent, which means you will sell faster and more!

If your trained eye immediately recognizes which eyeglass colors will suit the customer exactly, you can quickly make the customer happy with the glasses within a few minutes by showing two to three glasses.

At peak times, as in summer, for example, it was not unusual for me to serve two customers at the same time and, by quickly filtering the colours of the glasses in my mind, to present them with certain glasses that they were immediately satisfied with and bought within a few minutes.

It makes you as an optician much more professional, so that you will feel how customers trust your opinion within a few seconds.

This automatically attracts even more customers, as customers naturally want to be served by someone they already trust.

This is exactly what makes you as a salesperson in the ophthalmic industry so attractive for customers!

How do you actually recognize the warm skin types?

The easiest and quickest way to recognize people with warm skin types is by their freckles and/or natural red hair. People with this hair colour always have a warm skin tone and are often characterised by green, blue or light brown, almost beige eye colours.

Famous people are Prince Harry, Emma Stone, Boris Becker, Barbara Meier, Palina Rojinski or Ed Sheeran.

Red-haired people with blue or beige eyes can be divided into spring pen. Thus the warm colours of the spring palette suit them best.

Examples are Amber Heard or Ed Sheeran.

Red-haired people with green eyes are divided into autumn types, so that the warm colours of the autumn palette stand out best.

Examples are Palina Rojinski or Emma Stone.

In addition to the red-haired warm colour types that are easy to recognise, there are also the very rare blonde-haired people who like the warm colours of the spring table best. These are particularly characterised by a light, slightly golden and rather pale skin colour. In addition, these people have either very light beige or light blue eyes with mostly green and/or yellow rings on the iris. Examples are Matthias Schweighöfer, Ewan Mc Gregor, Angela Merkel and myself.

How do you recognize the cool skin types?

Cool skin types are very easy and quick to recognise by their dark, almost black hair colour.

Usually these types have a dark skin color or become dark quickly by the sun. Their eye color often captivates by a very dark brown or a dark blue. Rarely there are also black-haired people with green or grey eyes. People with these characteristics have the coolest colours of the winter palette.

Examples are Mel Gibson, Barack Obama, Jonny Depp, Demi Moore.

Winter types are the most common in the world. Then follow the summer types.

Summer types often have an ash blond light or ash brown light hair and mostly have blue, blue-green, rarely also grey or light brown tones.

Examples are Heidi Klum, Paul Walker and Ryan Gosling.

My tip to you, dear optician, is to learn the colour types by heart and as an exercise compare the pictures of the prominent colour types with each other again and again, which I cited as an example. Then try to divide the different people into colour types in your daily life and consider which colours definitely suit these people and which not at all.

Warm skin types are flattered by beige, orange or golden tones.

Cold skin types, on the other hand, have very good black, grey or silver tones. The typical white is also characteristic for them.

If you regularly go through the colour palettes of the four skin types, you will learn to get a feeling for what cold and warm colours are.

The colour palettes of the spring, summer, autumn and winter types can be found very easily via Google search. Print them out and place them in places where you want to match them.

Also during your next clothing purchase it is advisable to take the colour tables with you and to understand the classification into the colour types. You can practice the same with your eyewear assortment!

When you get new glasses, you should think about the colour types that these particular glasses can match. In this way you will be able to increase your professionalism and recommend the perfect glasses to the next customer in seconds!

Now that you have got to know all the important methods for successful consultation, you will learn in the next chapter how to start your perfect sales talk.

CHAPTER 12

HOW TO OPEN SALES TALKS FOR WHICH YOU WILL LOVE YOUR CUSTOMERS

"Failure is merely the possibility of starting smarter from scratch." ~ Henry Ford

In previous chapters you have already learnt how important it is to establish a friendly relationship with your customers so that they will be happy to buy glasses from you.

When a customer enters your store, it is very important how you start the conversation with him so that he immediately finds you sympathetic and at the same time gets involved in a sales conversation with you.

In this chapter you will get to know methods that make it easy for you to enter into a conversation with the customer and also arouse the customer's interest in a sales conversation.

How do you start a conversation?

When a customer enters your shop and first takes a look around, it is first and foremost your task to establish a sympathetic relationship with him.

Avoid sentences like: "Good day, you only look", "Hello, can I help you?" or "You wish?"

Instead, from now on you do it like sales professionals by applying the method praise and similarities.

Sales professionals in ophthalmic optics therefore first take a very close look at the new customer and look for something in him for which they can sincerely lobby him.

This could be, for example, a certain pair of glasses that the customer wears or a special hair colour that they simply find beautiful. Those who initially take this trouble as opticians will find things automatically and easily over time for which they can express their appreciation to other customers.

After you sincerely acknowledge the customer for a certain thing and he thanks you, you already create a good relationship with him, with which you can create a continuous conversation. In the following, you create similarities between you and your customer in order to create sympathy for each other. You remember that people prefer to be advised by like-minded people, which is why the opinion of friends has a high value.

What is the best way to find community?

Let's take the example by recognizing the customer's glasses. For example, you praise the great design and determine the fashionable style of the glasses.

As a common feature, you can then imagine that you, like your customer, have an affinity for the style of eyewear mentioned and, for example, also have experience with eyewear of this style.

If you now create a sympathetic conversation with your customer, then he or she will also be open to your ideas and suggestions, which you will recommend to him or her in the next step.

Next, initiate your sales talk by creating a gallant transition to your glasses.

Ask questions such as: "How does it sound to you if you try out our glasses in your own style?", "...which glasses can we inspire you with today?" or "Since you are coming to visit us today, what would you like to try?".

The aim of these questions is to prepare the customer for the next step and to prepare him mentally for buying glasses. Therefore, you are welcome to suggest that the next step is to look at glasses, take them in your hand or look at yourself with them in the mirror. Use the techniques of the previous chapters to inspire the customer and convince him of your competence.

Therefore, mirror your customers in facial expressions, gestures and posture. Use words that address his preferred sensory channel. Consult him according to his colour type and justify your choice of glasses.

Put the advantages of glasses in the foreground and only briefly mention the features. Identify the customer type in order to convince him only with his special buying motives. Give your customers an overview of your eyeglass selection by using the 3 glasses technique and ask targeted questions to ultimately lead the customer to a purchase.

In the next chapter you will find out which questions lead the customer to his purchase decision and when exactly you use them.

CHAPTER 13

KNOW BUY SIGNALS, USE DEAL TECHNIQUES AND SELL!

"Don't be afraid to give up the good to achieve the great!"
~ *John D. Rockefeller*

How many times have you experienced the following?

You see yourself with your customer in a pleasant glasses consultation, your customer likes to talk to you and lets you show him many glasses that could be interesting for him.

In the course of your conversation, however, there comes a point when your customer wants to say goodbye to you politely, seems unclosed and would like to take a look at something at alternative opticians in the city or on the Internet.

What happened here?

When a customer comes into your shop and looks around, even gets into a conversation with you and spends time with you, then your customer already gives you three buying signals!

A customer enters your shop because there is something that interests him. First buy signal! Therefore, treat a new customer with the greatest appreciation you can provide. An attentive "Welcome" puts the customer in the right mood here.

The customer gets into a conversation with you about glasses.

Second buy signal! Take the customer and his wishes very seriously and listen to the customer intensively in order to value his wishes.

Your customer also spends time in your shop, is shown glasses and holds a conversation with you. Third purchase signal!

So if you don't sell glasses to the customer towards the end, then from now on you will always take responsibility for them yourself. Why? It is largely up to you to find out more of the customer's purchase signals, to ask questions about the deal and to sell him the glasses.

Who can carry out the latter three tasks? That's right, you. This is exactly why you have an enormous influence on whether your customer buys or not.

How do you use final exam questions in the future?

Let's assume that your customer wants black plastic glasses with lenses for his nearsightedness. You then ask him how high his values are or whether you are allowed to measure his previous values? The customer agrees and lets you measure his previous glasses.

Secondly, you ask the customer in which situation he will wear his desired glasses?

Will they be everyday glasses, glasses only for the computer or rather fashionable leisure glasses?

How satisfied is he with his existing glasses and what benefits should his new glasses provide to make him completely satisfied?

Let the customer talk and repeat his answers in his own words. Furthermore, you ask them when they need the new glasses and lenses? The customer probably answers, "As quickly as possible, of course".

What happened next in the course of this conversation? You asked the customer the open questions (beginning with: What?, How?, With what?, When?, Which?, How many?) so that the customer would first tell you about his wishes. The customer unconsciously becomes aware of what he actually wants and you guide him more and more to a purchase decision through exactly this question structure.

Especially with the last open final question, when does he need the new glasses?

Your conversation now continues as follows after you have selected two black glasses for the customer:

You show the customer your two or three selected black glasses. You go through the 3 glasses rule and the benefit communication (as described in the previous chapters). Then you ask him whether he prefers the glasses with the strong or the thin frame, for example?

He chooses the thin frame. You would like to know whether he would like for example self-tinting glasses or rather classic glasses for a clear view without reflections in the glass? Your customer chooses the latter type of glass.

What have you now witnessed with your customer?

Your customer decides by your chosen alternative questions already unconsciously for a certain type of glasses. This will make your customer's purchase decision much easier and more tangible, especially because the customer will put together his desired glasses piece by piece.

Your sales talk will now culminate in the conclusion of the sale:

In the following, you will also ask the customer alternative questions in which the first option A in the question is the one that you want most for the customer and for yourself.

The latter option B may also constitute a possible additional sale. It is important that the customer independently makes a certain purchase decision for one or at best both options.

A question here can be whether the customer only wants black glasses (option A), or whether he also likes sunglasses (option B) for car journeys and the like? Now your customer decides for one or both glasses and you have indirectly a sales conclusion.

In order to finally sell the glasses to the customer, ask two more questions, the following as an example:

1. You can pick up your desired glasses, with your chosen lenses and the corresponding extras already this Friday completely made. How does that sound to you? (Alternatives: How do you see it? What do you think?)

The customer answers in the best case that it sounds good, or asks if necessary still further questions, which you answer to him.

2. Would you like to pick up your glasses in the morning or rather in the evening?

This is the last alternative question that you ask the customer as a final question, since he now decides on one of the two appointments and indirectly confirms the purchase.

In the end you create the purchase contract, tell him the price and ask him for his signature as well as for the payment.

If you read this chapter several times and prepare various closing questions for your consultation in advance, then practice this procedure as often as possible. If you have internalized this guideline in the sales talk, you will help in the future more courageously and more consistently your customers to make a purchase decision, so that these can save time and trouble.

And please remember, if you don't lead the customer to a purchase decision, another optician will take it over.

So, dear reader, draw a lot from the knowledge and experience of this book! Strive every day for your goals and implement new insights so that you achieve what you want. I wish you only the best!

VERIFICATIONS

1 Cf. Frank Bettger, Live enthusiastically and win, p. 30 ff.

2 Cf. Robert B. Cialdini, The Psychology of Persuasion, p. 44 ff.

3 Quoted after: Frank Bettger, Living ghosts and winning, p. 22.

4 Cf. Dr. Hans Georg Häusel, Brain Script, p. 89 ff.

5 Cf. Dr. Hans Georg Häusel, Brain Script, p. 119 ff.

6 Cf. Dr. Hans Georg Häusel, Brain Script, p. 119 ff.

7 Cf. Dr. Hans Georg Häusel, Brain Script, p. 119 ff.

8 Cf. Dr. Hans Georg Häusel, Brain Script, p. 119 ff.

9 Cf. Robert B. Cialdini, The Psychology of Persuasion, p. 36 ff.

10 Cf. Robert B. Cialdini, The Psychology of Persuasion, p. 44 ff.

NOTES

www.ingramcontent.com/pod-product-compliance
Lightning Source LLC
Chambersburg PA
CBHW030948240526
45463CB00016B/2067